Treating Cuts and Bruises

A Book on Wound Care

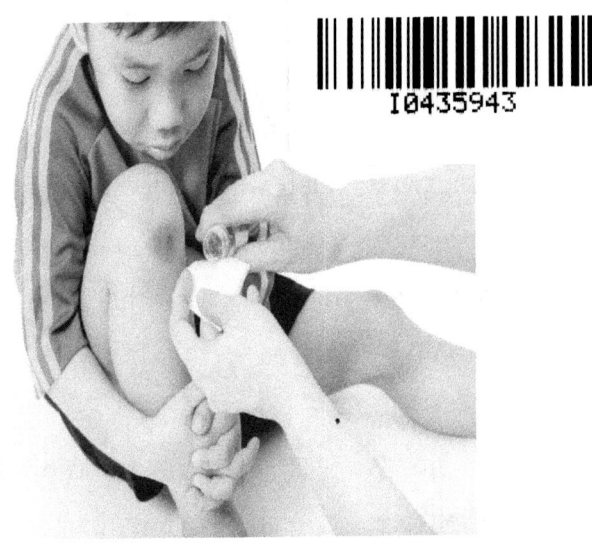

I0435943

By
Paolo Jose de Luna

Paolo Jose de Luna

The information provided herein is stated to be truthful and consistent, in that any liability, in terms of inattention or otherwise, by any usage or abuse of any policies, processes, or directions contained within is the solitary and utter responsibility of the recipient reader. Under no circumstances will any legal responsibility or blame be held against the publisher for any reparation, damages, or monetary loss due to the information herein, either directly or indirectly.

Respective authors own all copyrights not held by the publisher.

Paolo Jose de Luna

The information herein is offered for informational purposes solely, and is universal as so. The presentation of the information is without contract or any type of guarantee assurance.

The trademarks that are used are without any consent, and the publication of the trademark is without permission or backing by the trademark owner. All trademarks and brands within this book are for clarifying purposes only and are the owned by the owners themselves, not affiliated with this document.

Table of Contents

Introduction

At one point in life, every one of us has gotten a wound at least once or twice. Yes, getting wounded might be painful, but it's considered as the normal course of life. There are a number of reasons why we get wounded – both physically and emotionally. But in this book, we'll be focusing on the physical wounds that we get from time to time.

A wound is a type of injury, either occurring externally or internally on the body tissues, that serves as evidence of the damage that has occurred to the cells. Wounds often occur on the skin because the skin serves as the physical first line of defense against trauma and thus, cell damage. However, a strong enough amount of force can damage the skin, resulting in a variety of wounds depending on the type of injury that had occurred. There are a number of reasons as to how we get wounds – falls, cuts, small tools, sharp objects, and accidents.

For serious accidents or severe cases of wound or bleeding, you need to call your local emergency hotline so that you can get immediate medical attention. You can also ask a family member to bring you to the nearest hospital so you can get immediate medical attention, especially in the cases of severe wounds.

The usual concern for wounds is the risk for infection. Because wounds are open, they serve as the entry for bacteria which can cause infections. If you don't know how to properly clean and treat your wounds, you might be at risk for developing an infection. And everyone knows that infections are more serious and they can further increase your spending since you'll need to get antibiotics to fight off the infection on top of the materials that you need in order to take care of your wounds. Sometimes, you may need to get hospitalized to fight off a serious case of infection that had occurred on a particular wound. Worst case scenario, the infection on a wound reaches the roof of severity and a surgeon may need to surgically cut off dead infected tissue or even cut off a part of the body like finger, hand, or leg.

In this book, you'll be learning all about wounds. This will include the different types of wounds, the signs and symptoms of each type of wound, how to properly take care of different wounds, the common management in taking care of wounds, the myths and hoaxes surrounding wound care, and the common remedies that you can use to treat different kinds of wounds. You'll be presented with a number of facts regarding wounds and wound care that will help you understand how to identify each type of wound, eliminating the risk of complications through untrained and unproven methods on wound care, how to differentiate each type of wound from each other, and how to treat each type of wound properly with careful and utmost care.

So, get a pen and paper to take some notes and better be ready with your first aid kits, bandages, and antiseptic sprays – it's time to learn more about wounds and wound care.

Chapter 1 - What are Wounds?

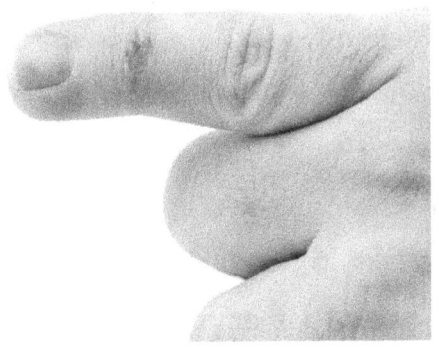

A wound is a type of injury that can either be internal or external in nature which indicates a break or damage in the body tissues, usually the skin since it serves as the first line of defense against physical trauma. At one way or another, almost everyone will experience getting wounded some time in their life. Most wounds are often minor and can easily be treated at home, usually by cleaning the wound with water, applying some antiseptic, and putting adhesive plaster or Band-Aid for most people.

There are a lot of reasons as to why people can get wounded. Some get wounded from falling, some get wounded from sharp objects around the house like knives in the kitchen, an exposed sharp end of a nail on a wooden plank, or even just the sharp edge of a furniture. In the more serious cases, car accidents, displays of violence, animal attacks, friction, or even heat. In some cases, these wounds can be so serious that you may need to seek medical attention immediately to prevent the development of complications. Wounds that have a lot of bleeding or if the bleeding goes on for too long, you need to see a doctor right away or you might just be asking for the inevitable worst.

Different Types of Wounds

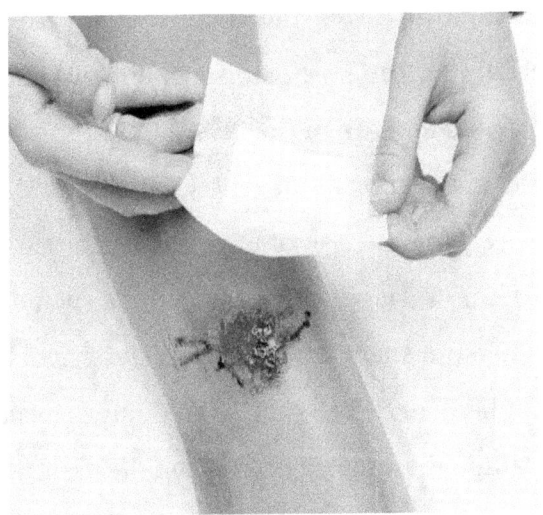

Now that you know the basics about wounds, it's time to know the different types of wounds that you can get throughout your lifetime. First off, wounds can be separated into two main classifications – <u>open wounds</u> and <u>closed wounds</u>.

By definition, an open wound is a type of injury that may cause an internal or external break in the body tissues, often occurring on the skin. Open wounds provide a break in the cell membrane and creates a portal of entry for bacteria, increasing the risk of infection to develop. Common causes of open wounds include cuts from sharp objects, excessive friction applied on the skin, and blunt force trauma that manages to break the skin.

There are five (5) types of open wounds, namely: abrasions, incisions, avulsions, lacerations, and punctures. Each type of open wound has their own shape and has their own way to treat them properly.

- **Incisions** – Resulting from a cut, usually from a sharp object like a blade, a knife, or a piece of broken glass, an incision is a type of open wound that can cause a lot of bleeding and these wounds bleed quickly. Incisions often aren't that serious since they're commonly shallow wounds that only extend to the skin and the epidermis. However, a deep incision may cause damage to the ligaments, tendons, muscles, or even cut a major blood vessel.

- **Lacerations** – This type of open wound is deeper compared to that of an incision, tearing the topmost layer of the skin and extending to the epidermis or the thick chunk of tissue under the skin. Common

15

causes of lacerations come from mishandling sharp tools like knives and machines. A lacerated wound's bleeding is more rapid and much more extensive compared to light incisions or abrasions.

- **Abrasions** – This type of open wound often occurs when the skin rubs against a rough surface, resulting from the excessive amount of friction on the soft and delicate skin, causing the skin to peel off and damage the overall structure of the tissues and the blood vessels. A good example of an abrasion would be a road rash and a lesser type of abrasion would be from tripping on the ground. When it comes to abrasions, there isn't much blood, but the wound still needs to be cleaned properly to avoid infection from developing and setting in.

- **Avulsions** – When the skin and tissue tears away due to an extensive amount of force, an avulsion is made. This type of open wound occurs in cases like vehicular accidents, explosions, crushing incidents, animal bites, and gunshots. Victims of avulsion tend to breathe quite heavily and they bleed profusely. If you have an avulsion or if you see someone with an avulsion, call 911 or your local medical emergency team immediately to get medical help. If those with avulsion don't get treated in time, they might die from cardiac arrest or from severe bleeding.

- **Punctures** – Characterized as a small hole in the skin, a puncture is an open wound caused by a long, sharp, and pointed object like a needle, a bullet, an ice pick, or a nail. Though smaller in size and they may not bleed much, a puncture is considered to be a grave wound because of how far it can reach inside the body. For example, an ice pick or a bullet can reach as far as the lungs or the heart, extensively damaging vital organs. If you have a puncture wound, even if it's just a small wound like stepping on a rusty nail, go and visit your physician immediately to get a booster shot for tetanus and prevent the development of infection which is quite common among those who have puncture wounds and refrained from seeking medical attention.

On the other hand, closed wounds are wounds that don't cause a break in the skin and the surrounding area of the wound is not exposed. The usual cause of a closed wound is blunt force trauma or from accidents which often results in a bruise or swelling in an area – both signs of damaged blood vessels and tissues underneath the skin.

However, don't take closed wounds for granted even though the injury is little to be seen – the damage can be more extensive compared to open wounds and may even reach internal organs, putting the life of the victim in danger. Here are the different types of closed wounds that you should know about.

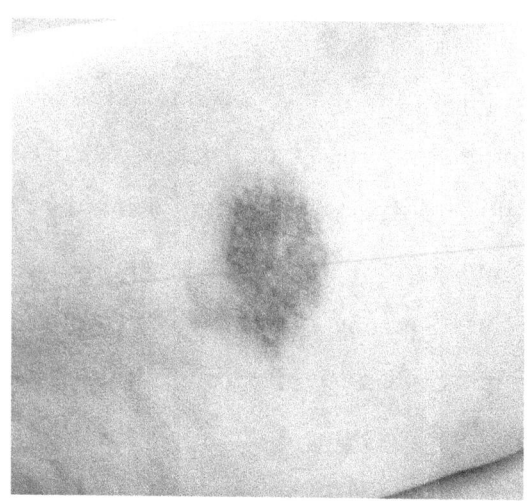

- **Hematomas** – This type of closed wound results from the damage to the small blood vessels, causing blood to spill out from the blood vessels and collecting into the interstitial spaces in the tissues. This later becomes a soft and spongy lesion or lump on the affected area, displaying a change in color depending on how severe the injury is. Hematomas are painful and they can vary in size and depth, depending on its severity.

- **Contusions** – A common type of sports injury, a contusion results from a direct application of blunt force trauma to an area of the body, resulting in the damage to the small blood vessels, the muscles, the ligaments, some of the internal organs, and sometimes even the bones. Contusions appear as reddish to bluish bruises on the area which then spreads over the injured area. Ice compress is a common first aid method for those who have suffered from a contusion. Though fairly common and easy to treat, a contusion can vary in how severe it can become depending on the area affected. For example, a contusion on the skull is considered as a medical emergency because the brain can get damaged.

- **Crush Injuries** – Resulting from a high amount of pressure that squeezes an area of the body, crush injuries are pretty self-explanatory. Trapped between two surfaces, a part of the body (most usually a limb) suffers damaged from the force. The damage from a crush injury can vary depending on the weight of the area of the body and the crushing object that caused the injury in the first place. Crush injuries can show varying degrees from a small bruise up to the complete damage of the area, even crushing bone into tiny little pieces as shown in a comminuted fracture.

Knowing the various types of wounds is essential if you want to know how to treat each one. Getting to know the basics about wounds is important in providing treatment and preventing complications from developing. Different types of wounds require different medical treatment methods which we'll talk about in the succeeding chapters of this book.

Chapter 2 - Developing a Keen Eye

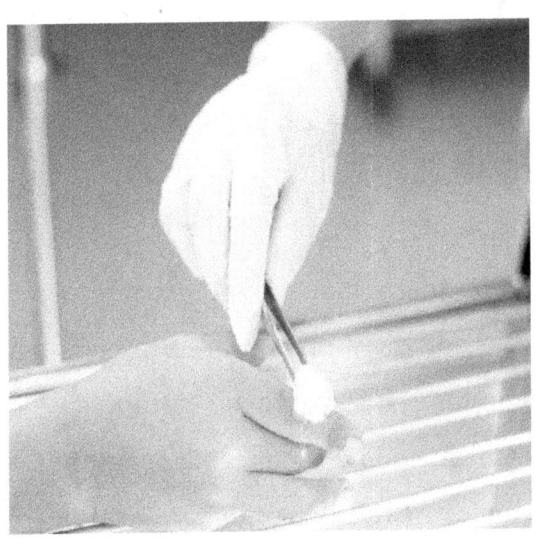

It's one thing knowing the different types of wounds. But it's much more difficult to develop a keen and discerning eye that can differentiate any kind of wound from other types and applying the appropriate measures to treat it properly. You don't want to embarrass yourself by applying a cold compress on an avulsed type of wound. With the wrong interventions and the wrong assessment of the wound, you can actually make the injury even worse. Here are the things that you should take note of when it comes to identifying wounds.

While there may be different types of wounds, there are common signs and symptoms that you need to take note of. Here are some signs and symptoms of wounds that you should learn to identify.

- Pain
- Swelling or inflammation
- Redness on the affected area
- Bleeding
- Tearing of the skin
- Bruising

Wound Infections

But aside from the common signs and symptoms of wounds, you also need to take note of the common complication of wounds – infection. When it comes to wounds, infections are quite serious. Aside from cleaning the wound, you need to treat the infection that has just set in with antibiotics. Knowing how to tell if an infection has set in on the wound is critical since this is considered as a case that needs immediate medical intervention. If you notice any of the following signs, see your attending physician as soon as possible to treat the infection and prevent further damage on the wound.

- The wound becomes increasingly more reddish
- The wound becomes more painful

- When a yellowish or greenish fluid starts to drain from the wound
- When the wound starts to develop a rancid smell
- If you develop a fever
- You have a faster heart rate
- You have a decreased blood pressure
- When you have swelling lymph nodes

When you see any of these signs and symptoms, don't hesitate to go to your doctor right away. Most probably, you'll have to start an antibiotic to treat the infection depending on the microorganism that has infected your wound. If the infection is severe, you'll have to be admitted in a hospital and antibiotics administered through your veins or introduced intravenously should be done to treat the infection as soon as possible. If your doctor finds that the infection is still manageable at an out-patient or home care basis, then you're probably going to be prescribed with antibiotics that may come in forms of tablets, capsules, or syrups for children.

Tetanus

Aside from infection, *tetanus* is another serious complication of wounds. Also known as lockjaw, this type of infection brings about severe muscle spasms that affects the jaw, the limbs, and even the airway muscles, leading to a fatal result if medical intervention is not done immediately. In tetanus, the muscle spasms last from a few seconds up to several minutes, putting the person's life in danger since it can halt breathing if not managed appropriately.

If you're still not convinced on how deadly tetanus is, the spasms that occur are so strong that it can even shatter bones. Other signs and symptoms that you need to watch out for include the following:

- Fever
- Excessive sweating
- Headache
- Sensitivity to light
- Difficulty in swallowing
- Increased blood pressure
- Increased heart rate

Symptoms usually appear 3 to 21 days after the infection occurs. The recovery, on the other hand, is quite long – ranging from weeks to even months to completely recover. However, 10% of those with tetanus die from complications like the spasm of the airway which warrants the need for an immediate surgical procedure, a tracheostomy tube insertion.

While the first thing on a medical practitioner's mind when they encounter patients experiencing difficulty or a complete halt of breathing is to insert a endotracheal tube to provide an artificial airway, that's not the case for those with tetanus. The muscles surrounding the airway experience severe spasm which makes an intubation useless since the airway closes and blocks the entry of air. A tracheostomy tube insertion is often warranted as an artificial airway is surgically inserted directly into the trachea for airway entry.

The primary culprit in tetanus is *Clostridium tetani*, a bacteria that can be found in soil, dust, and animal waste. This bacteria can cause an infection by entering a break in the skin like wounds, specifically through punctures and cuts due to a sharp object like an exposed nail, a needle, or a sharp tool. Clostridium tetani then produces a toxin which causes the muscles to stop contracting properly.

Chapter 3 - The How-To's of Wound Care

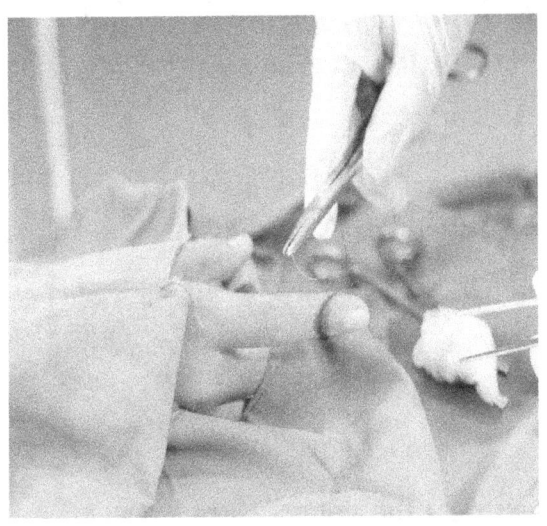

Taking care of a wound isn't all that difficult. However, it's actually easier said than done. While it can be done by anyone, taking care of a wound requires knowledge, skill, and materials to ensure that the wound stops bleeding and infection doesn't set in. After knowing more about the different types of wounds, the complications of wounds like infection and tetanus, and all the basics about wounds, it's time to know how to take care of wounds properly and efficiently.

First off, there are things that you should remember when it comes to taking care of wounds. There are things that you should and shouldn't do as there are a lot of people who end up doing the wrong things for the right reasons when it comes to tending to their wounds. Most often, they end up with a slow healing or even an infected wound. Here are the things that you should and shouldn't do when it comes to wound care.

Treating Cuts and Bruises

What you should NOT do:

- Don't use alcohol on open wounds. The intense burning sensation of cleansing alcohol is so strong.

- Don't stay too long under the sun. Ultraviolet rays of the sun can hinder in the healing process of the wounds.

- Don't ignore changing dressings for the wound. This can promote infection and prevent healing of the wound.

- Don't apply things like toothpaste, butter, oil, or other foreign substances that may be recommended by other people. These are only speculated to work based only on their personal beliefs, but there are no medical evidences that these substances work. In fact, applying some of these substances can make the wound even worse, preventing it from healing or even causing infection.

- Don't scratch the wound. Scratching can reopen the wound and can the bleeding even worse.

- Don't try to expose the wound to air. Cover it with a Band-Aid or an adhesive to protect it from dirt and debris. This also protects the wound from getting infected.

- Don't try to pick off the scab. These hard and often unsightly remains of a healing wound protect the wound from dirt and dust, preventing the incidence of infection.

- Don't put anything like butter, ointments, or toothpaste on a burn wound. Burn wounds are unique and they need to be cooled down with cool running water. If the burn is extensive and extremely painful, you should go to a hospital to have it checked out.

- Don't use contaminated or dirty water to clean your wounds. While it's important to wash the wound, using contaminated water will increase the risk of infecting the wound and you can even get sick once the contaminated water enters the wound.

What you SHOULD do:

- Clean your wound with clean running water and soap to cleanse it from bacteria and debris. This will prevent infection from setting in and also aids in the healing process of the wound.
- Apply gentle pressure on the wound with a clean cloth or dressing. This will reduce the bleeding and help in minimizing the injury while the wound heals naturally.
- Dress an open wound with povidone iodine. This dark brown solution is an antiseptic that promotes healing and prevents bacterial infection on various types of wounds. It has become a

staple for medical practitioners to use povidone iodine in treating several kinds of wounds. It's gentle to the nerves and won't cause pain when applied to the wound.

- Wash your hands with water and cleanse with 70% isopropyl alcohol before and after handling the wound. This will prevent the wound from being contaminated and prevent you from spreading all the germs around.

- Remove a Band-Aid or a dressing on the wound slowly as this lowers the risk of removing the scab and reopening the wound. If your dressing is tied down with plaster, rubbing it with a cotton ball dampened with alcohol can help removing it much easier.

- See your doctor immediately if the wound is extensive or doesn't stop bleeding. This means that the wound may need medical intervention to heal properly and prevent infection.

When to See Your Doctor

Most people fear of going to the doctor, that's why most of us tend to turn to common knowledge or surfing the net for solutions when it comes to taking care of wounds. However, there are times when you should have your wound checked out by a health professional. Here are the things that you should watch out for your wounds to tell you that you should seek medical consultation.

- The wound is too large or extensive. This may need to be sutured up in the emergency room. Large wounds on the face may even need to be repaired cosmetically.

- The wound is deep (about ½ inch up to 1 inch). This means that the object that may have caused the wound may have injured an internal organ. Have yourself checked out to make sure that you don't have other complications.

- The bleeding doesn't stop with direct pressure or by elevating the wound. You may need the wound to have stitched up and you may need to be given medications that help in promoting your blood to clot for the wound to heal up properly.

- The bleeding continues for more than 15 minutes. Bleeding this long can warrant the need for blood transfusion, especially when it's because of an accident or a traumatic injury.

- A wound coming from a serious accident like a car accident needs to be checked out immediately. This is to rule out other complications and to see that other organs in the body are undamaged from the accident.

- Wounds from animal bites also need to be checked out. Animals harbor various germs in their mouth and it can easily cause infection. Snake bites from venomous snakes need some antitoxin while insect bites from bees or wasps may need the administration of epinephrine to counteract the inflammatory reaction of the body. Bites from mammals like dogs, cats, raccoons, and squirrels may need you to have a booster shot for rabies along with tetanus boosters. Animal bites have a higher chance to get infected, so better consult with your physician immediately.

- An infected wound that has pus or redness around the area should be checked out by your doctor. A small infection coming from a cut can lead to a serious infection and contaminate your whole body, resulting in sepsis or infection of the blood, if you don't get immediate medical attention.

Materials for Wound Care

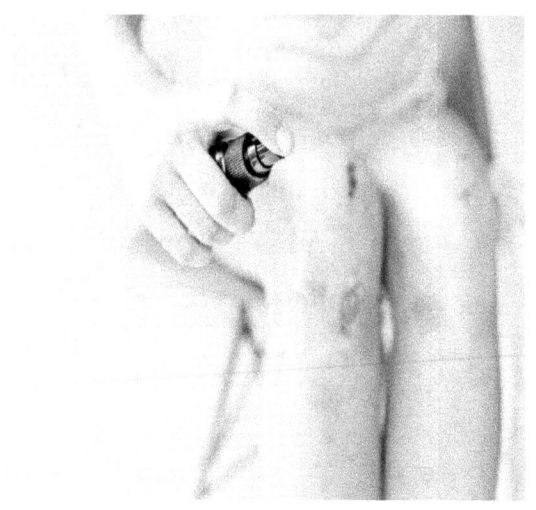

Before starting to tend to your wounds, you need to be properly equipped with the right materials. Most often, you can get these materials in your local drug store or pharmacy. In fact, you can gather these materials and shove them in a box to create your own first aid kit at home! First aid of a wound is quick and easy if you know what to do and you have the right materials.

- Adhesives or plasters (ex. Band-Aid, Micropore, Leukoplast)
- Cotton balls
- 70% isopropyl alcohol
- Povidone iodine (ex. Betadine solution)
- Sterile gauze pad of different sizes.
- Wound cleansing spray
- Cotton applicators
- Ice compress or ice pack (for closed wounds)

How to Dress Your Wound

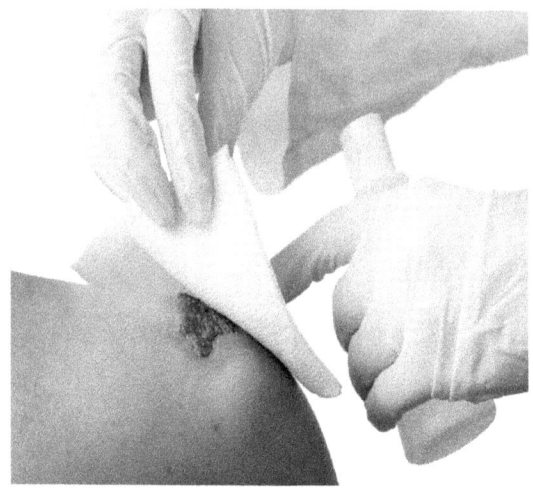

Dressing a wound is easy once you know how to do it and you have the right materials for the job. Most wounds are treated at home and often don't need to be checked by a physician. Here are the steps that you can take in order to treat your wounds at home.

- Clean your hands with soap and water. You can also use 70% isopropyl alcohol to cleanse your hands before and after you treat a wound, whether it's your own or someone else's wounds. This will prevent the contamination of a wound and prevent the spread of infection.

- Clean the wound with clean running water and soap to remove the debris and germs from the wound. This cleanses the wound and prevents infection. Small wounds can immediately be covered with a small dressing or a Band-Aid to keep the wound dry and protected from germs.

- For a closed wound, apply an ice compress and elevate the wound. This will reduce the swelling and allow the affected area to rest for a while.

- For an open wound, control bleeding by applying direct pressure on the wound. If possible, you should use both of your hands and firmly apply direct pressure on the wound for a few minutes. This will reduce bleeding and give the wound time to close up and heal naturally.

- Elevate the site of bleeding above the heart. This will reduce the blood flow towards the wound and helps in stopping the bleeding. Most wounds stop bleeding for about 10 minutes and can be applied with a dressing over the wound thereafter.

- Once you've controlled the bleeding, you can now proceed to dress the wound by using a sterile gauze pad to cover the wound while still applying direct pressure to the wound.

- If the sterile gauze pad you've applied on the wound is soaked, replace it with a new one. If the wound still continues bleeding, apply another gauze pad on top of it instead. A thick slab of gauze pad helps control the bleeding along with direct pressure.

- At this point, you can apply povidone iodine to the wound by using a cotton ball or cotton applicator. Spread it thoroughly on and around the wound. This prevents infection to set in and promotes the healing of the wound. Povidone iodine like Betadine is gentle to the wound and isn't painful when applied directly to the wound.

- Cover the wound with a dry sterile gauze pad. Make sure to keep it firmly, but not too tightly to allow the wound to have some breathing room. This ensures that there is still adequate circulation of blood to the site.

- Put the gauze in place with an adhesive like a plaster. For a tight and ensure fit, use a Leukoplast plaster – the brown adhesive plaster that provides a strong stick to the skin. But if you're allergic to

Leukoplast or any of its variants, you can use a much friendlier plaster like Transpore or Micropore.

- For deeper wounds, applying direct pressure and dressing it with a sterile gauze pad is enough since they can be painful when you clean them.

- Dress the wound on a regular basis and everyday by using the previous steps mentioned here. This is to ensure that the wound heals properly and infection is prevented from ever happening.

- Check your wound frequently for any signs of infection. This would include things like redness, swelling, a foul smell, discharges, pus, or the wound doesn't heal altogether.

You shouldn't be scared of treating a wound. Knowing how to take care of a wound is essential since you'll be treating most cuts and bruises at home. With the right materials at home, building your very own first aid kit is important for any family and you can be sure that you'll be using it eventually. But always remember that don't overestimate yourself and **seek medical attention** if your wound seems to be out of the ordinary like when it's infected or if a closed wound seems to have hit a vital area of your body. Keep your composure and don't hesitate to call for help when you really need it.

Conclusion

Treating Wounds Made Easy

The sight of blood can easily turn anyone off. If you're like most people who get all anxious and fearful upon seeing the bright scarlet color of blood, then know that you're not alone. However, you shouldn't let that stop you when it comes to treating your own injuries.

Wounds are quite common in our everyday lives. We can get it while cooking, working in the garage, gardening, or even just bumping into something around the house. Getting cut or bruised is quite common and you shouldn't be afraid of that. But you should learn how to properly treat these wounds at home since these kinds of injuries don't really need immediate medical attention and they're not even considered as an emergency case.

Knowing the different types of wounds that you can get, getting the right materials in taking care of a wound, and knowing the steps on how to treat a wound are essential when it comes to wound care.

Sure – at first it can look tough and difficult with all the medical knowledge that you'll be introduced. However, reading through and getting to know the twists and turns of wound care will make things a lot easier for you. Once you get the hang of it, treating wounds, whether it's your own or the wounds of others, can become quick, easy, and efficient as it can be.

www.ingramcontent.com/pod-product-compliance
Lightning Source LLC
Chambersburg PA
CBHW071250280526
45788CB00004B/1656